CW0390A866

SEX
GAMES

QUIVER

Contents

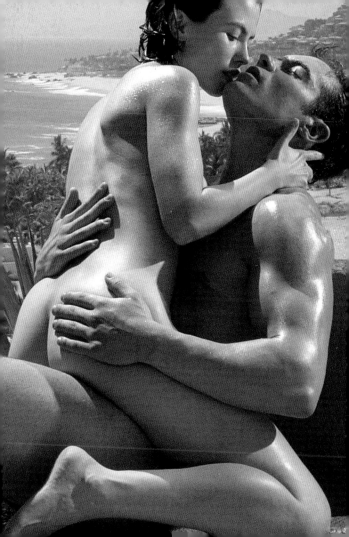

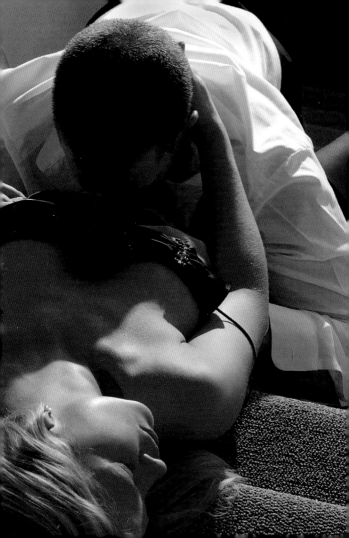

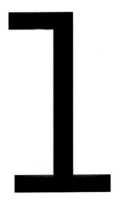

Stair Climber

Upstairs, downstairs—your stairs are
the perfect place for playing this game
of up and down (and in and out)!

The Sexy Setup

Leave or send your lover a suggestive note telling her to meet you on the staircase at a set time. Mention that you're dreaming of going up . . . and going down.

Rules & Tools

You should wear clothing that is easily removable: for women, a button-down shirt and zip-up skirt; for men, a button-down shirt and boxer shorts. If your stairs are not carpeted, bring out a blanket.

Playing the Game

Sweet and safe: In this version, you're (the stair "climber") in control. Have her position herself five or six stairs up, then tie one or both of her wrists to one of the banisters. Start at her toes and remove her clothing, piece by piece. You can be gentle and teasing, or get a little rough and tear or pull her clothes off. Once you come within range of her mouth, tease her by brushing your lips, belly, or penis near her face and mouth. Once she's naked, service her from your stairway position, either by spreading her legs for intercourse or having her open her mouth to suck you.

Hot and spicy: In this version, the stair climber is the slave, and you (positioned on the stairs) are the master. Position yourself three or four stairs up, completely naked, and direct your lover to start at your toes and climb, all the while licking, kissing, or exploring every inch of you. Once her face reaches your face take time to kiss passionately, but then ask her to go back down the stairs and repeat the process as needed. Your perch on the edge of the stair should give her the perfect position for exploring your manhood, but don't be afraid to grab her, position her at the edge of the stairs, and penetrate her fully.

Up the Ante

- Try either of the above games with your (or your lover's) backside facing outward.

- Blindfold the stair captive so she doesn't know what's coming next, then introduce a feather and massage oil for teasing her inner thighs, lower back, and nape of the neck.

- Move your lover to the laundry room: Have her hop on top of the washing machine or dryer and pull you into her. The vibrations will intensify every sensation!

- Pick her up and carry her, with you still inside her, to the pool table. Drive your shaft into her pocket!

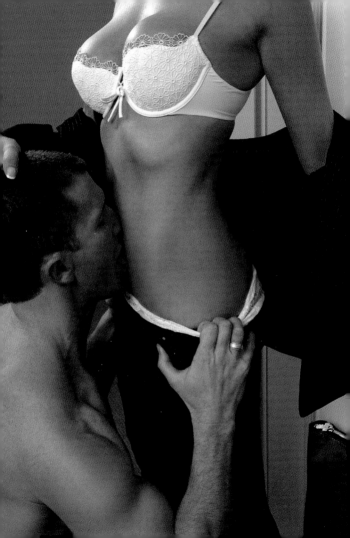

2

Strip Poker

How about a hand of cards, winner
takes all—or should we say,
winner takes *off* all?

Play to your lover's ego and mention you'd like to play strip poker, but you're sure *you'll* be the one doing most of the undressing.

Rules & Tools

Set a sexy scene, take out a deck of playing cards, and review the rules (see box). Figure out ahead of time how the game will work: For poker, each time you lose a hand you have to take off an article of clothing. Assemble a big pile of coins and divide it into two sets, one for each of you.

How to play seven-card stud poker: Deal two cards facedown and one card faceup. Make a bet (e.g., fifty cents, one dollar, etc.), then deal three cards faceup and the final card facedown. Winning hands (highest to lowest) are as follows: royal flush, straight flush, flush, full house, three of a kind, two pair, one pair. One pair beats the highest card in the hand.

Playing the Game

Sweet and safe: The winner of each hand gets to tell the other player which article of clothing to take off. See whether you can continue this drawn-out foreplay until one (or both) of you is fully undressed, then let the winner decide how he or she wants to be serviced. Consider setting satisfaction rules, such as only using your hands or your mouth.

Hot and spicy: The winner of each hand gets to command the loser to take off an article of clothing and perform a service, such as "massage my feet," "stroke my breasts," or "suck on the tip of my penis." Continue this drawn-out card play/foreplay until one of you is fully undressed. At this point, switch over to a fantasy game where your lover becomes a card shark and you're a gambler who has run out of money (or vice versa). The card shark gets to decide how you will pay off your debt, whether that means sucking him off or performing other services to his satisfaction.

Up the Ante

- Invite friends over for a group game of strip poker. Set some ground rules beforehand (unless you don't mind hosting a game of swap partners or swinging 101!).

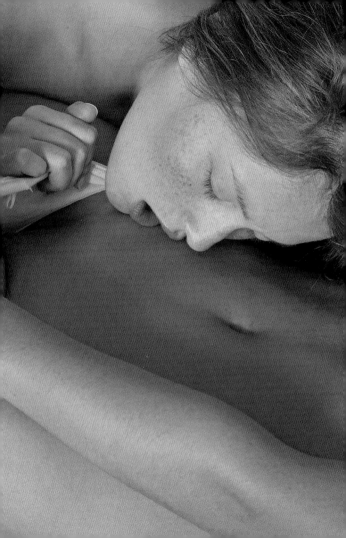

3

Naughty
Nap Time

Here's a naughty game that's
purrrrrfect for a lazy Sunday
afternoon at home.

The Sexy Setup

Write your lover a naughty note, spray it with a new fragrance or cologne, and leave it by his coffee or put it in his coat pocket. Write something like this: "Breathe in the scent of this note. Each time you smell this scent on me in the coming days you will have an uncontrollable desire to go into the bedroom and take a nap. Once you lie down, you are not allowed to open your eyes, speak, or use your hands, no matter what happens."

Rules & Tools

You can stick with your favorite scent of perfume or cologne (sweet and safe) or body lotion (hot and spicy) or, better yet, buy something new for the occasion—the sexier the better!

Playing the Game

Sweet and safe: Spray on your new scent and cuddle up to your lover. Ask him if he likes the smell, then remind him of your note. Give him a few minutes to get to the bedroom, then quietly enter the room. Be as quiet as possible as you blindfold and then undress your lover.

Kiss him all over; as your man gets excited, gently touch the area between his scrotum and anus, making him squirm for more. When the time is right, climb on top of him and bring him to orgasm.

Hot and spicy: Write the same type of note, but in addition to spraying it with perfume or cologne, also attach a small amount of lotion in a small plastic bag. Once your lover gets to the bedroom, warm up the lotion in your hands, then give him a sensual massage with plenty of teasing moves and loving caresses. When the time is right, lube up your hand (or fingers) and bring your lover to a wet and creamy orgasm.

Up the Ante

- Sign the note "Your Venus Butterfly." Then teach him how to perform this much talked about sexual technique: He should use his tongue on your clitoris, place several fingers in your vagina and use the other hand to stroke your buttocks or penetrate your anus. Be prepared for a multifaceted orgasm! (Women can perform a variation of this by sucking on his penis, cupping his testicles or stroking behind his balls with one hand, and slipping a finger into his anus with the other hand.)

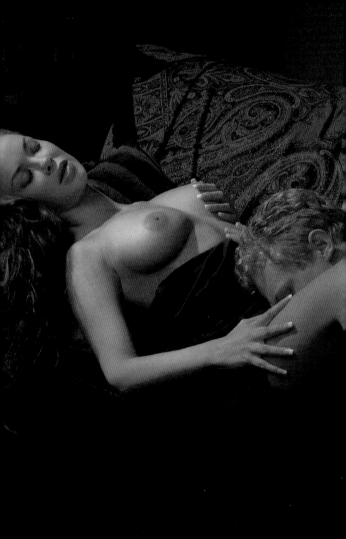

4

Blue Velvet

Nothing to do on a Saturday night?
Play this sweet and naughty game
of pain-and-pleasure using
your softest fabrics.

The Sexy Setup

Send your lover a note telling him about the special room in your house devoted to pleasure. In it, there's a bed of velvet and fake fur blankets. Your lover is invited to spend a few hours in this sensual heaven, with you as the mistress of erotic pleasure.

Rules & Tools

Assemble your softest, most sensual fabrics and focus on making your bed (or couch) a zone of pleasure for the skin. Make a quick trip to the fabric store and buy some velvet or velour castoffs to create a soft, velvety area for your lover to lie on, then pull out your softest cashmere sweater or wrap, silk scarves or gloves, fur accessories, a feather, and any other clothing or fabric that feels good on bare skin. When your lover arrives, blindfold him and lead him into the pleasure chamber. For the hot and spicy version of the game, be sure to have some ice cubes or a popsicle on hand.

Playing the Game

Sweet and safe: Use the various fabrics to touch his entire body. Slowly sweep the silk across his nipples, tease his inner thighs with a caress of velvet, and tickle his lower back with a brush of fur. Massage and caress your lover with each fabric, but avoid the genitals on purpose. Occasionally brush your nipples across his face, or lightly kiss his lower back. Eventually your travels lead you to massaging his penis with velvet-, fur-, or cashmere-covered hands.

Hot and spicy: Use one fabric at a time to stroke his penis and ask him to guess what each one is. If he gets it wrong, run an ice cube or Popsicle over his nipples, penis, or testicles for an exciting, icy jolt (make it quick, otherwise it might be painful. On the other hand, some lovers like mixing pain with pleasure . . .). If he guesses correctly, reward him with a deep, passionate kiss.

Up the Ante

- Tie your lover's hands together using a length of velvet or silk, then tease his neck, chest, nipples, belly, inner thighs, lower back, penis, or testicles with the other fabrics. Try to bring your lover to orgasm using just the touch of fabric—silk on the clitoris, and so on.

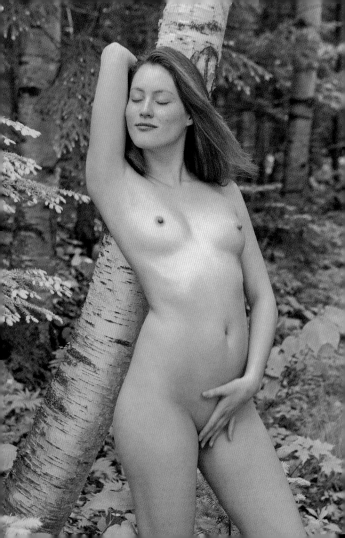

5

"Horny on Line One"

This is a great game for those nights when your lover is traveling on business or you're off on a girls' weekend at the spa.

The Sexy Setup

Tell your lover you need him to set aside some private time on the phone with you tonight—clothing optional, of course. Alternatively, get his juices flowing by leaving an erotic voice mail, email, or text message.

Rules & Tools

If you need to, practice your sultry, sexy voice beforehand. You might also want to learn some new erotic lingo for describing his body parts and yours. Before you dial, dim the lights, sip some wine, or look at some erotic pictures to get your juices flowing. Tell your lover anything goes, including pleasuring himself while you talk. Have your vibrator on hand, too.

Playing the Game

Sweet and safe: First time having phone sex? Try an opening line like "I wish you were lying here with me." Then proceed to tell him what you're wearing, how it feels to slip off each piece of clothing, or how your erect nipples feel to your own fingers. The goal is to paint him a picture that's alluring and erotic.

Ask him questions, such as "Do you want to kiss my nipples?" or "Do you want to feel how wet I'm getting?" Start touching yourself, and describe every effect and sensation—your erect nipples, your soft skin, your tingling clitoris. Bring yourself to orgasm, and don't forget the sound effects: Soft moans, sighs of pleasure, throaty groans, or heavy breathing can add to the pleasure!

Hot and spicy: Tell him to get naked and begin stroking himself. As he touches himself, tell him you're imagining what his penis feels like, how hard and large he is, and what an incredibly sexy man he is. As he begins to get turned on, describe what you'd be doing if you were there—kissing his chest, licking his shaft, rubbing his buttocks, or sucking his testicles. As he brings himself to orgasm, urge him on and tell him how hot he's making you. Then turn up your vibrator and let him listen in on the action while you get off!

Up the Ante

- Ask your lover how he would feel if you tied his hands together, if you and a friend ganged up on him together, or if he'd like you to try something different, like anal penetration. Then go on to describe the situation that turns him on the most.

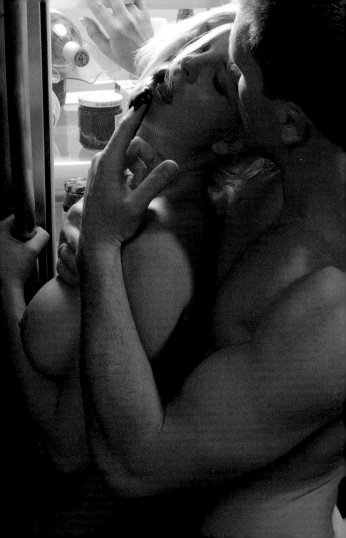

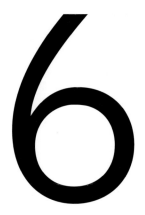

6

Make Me Your Own Sundae

Dessert's on me—literally! Let your lover build
his own sundae using you as the dish.

The Sexy Setup

Mention there's something special in the works for dessert, and he better get home before everything melts. The menu includes mountains of luscious whipped cream, gooey chocolate syrup, creamy caramel sauce, sweetened maraschino cherries, firm, peeled bananas—and, of course, *you*!

Rules & Tools

Have all of the "menu" items ready and just before your lover comes into the room, sit naked on the counter, dip a finger into the chocolate, and spread your legs seductively.

Playing the Game

Sweet and safe: Hand feed him cherries, let him lick chocolate off your fingers, and smear whipped cream on your belly. Then ask him to follow the trail of caramel leading downward with his tongue . . .

Hot and spicy: Dip your nipples in melted chocolate, outline your breasts in whipped cream, smear caramel on your inner thighs, and put a cherry in your belly button. Use this command: *Devour me!*

Up the Ante

- Hide the cherry between your legs and ask your lover to find it.

- Cover your clitoris with whipped cream and have him lick it off.

- Masturbate with the banana (while he watches) and have him eat the remains.

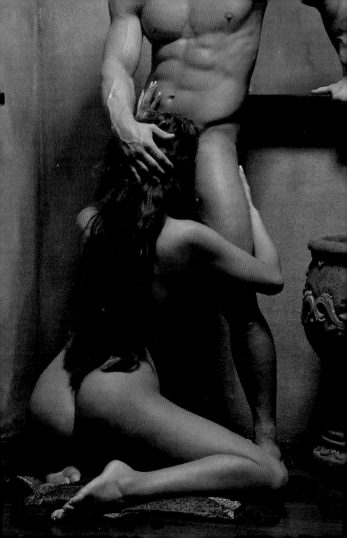

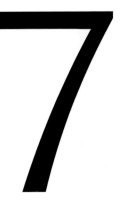

7

Peppermint Tingler

Use the flavor of mint to spice up your
sex life with this erotic game.

The Sexy Setup

Tell your lover you've planned a minty game with plenty of cool sensations.

Rules & Tools

Buy your favorite flavor of Altoid mints. Pour two glasses of peppermint schnapps, or, if you don't drink, a small glass of cinnamon or minty mouthwash.

Playing the Game

Sweet and safe: Chew some of the Altoids before giving your lover a blow job, or ask your lover to eat Altoids before going down on you. The tingling sensation you feel in your mouth when you chew these mints will intensify the sensation of oral sex for your partner.

Hot and spicy: Tip your glasses to one another and take a small sip of the schnapps. Run your tongues around one another's lips, then slowly move your mouth down your lover's body, leaving a minty cool trail across his skin. Ask your lover to circle your nipples with his minty tongue. Let it pool in your belly button, and then have him lap it out.

Trace a path all the way to his penis. Once you reach your lover's genitals, take another small sip—just enough so that you don't swallow it or drop a whole mouthful over your sweetie's privates. As you slip your mouth over his penis, let the liqueur or mouthwash drip down his shaft. The tingly sensation will drive him wild. If your lover does the same to you, tell him to be especially careful when letting the liqueur drip onto your clitoris and labia, and never let the liqueur or mouthwash get inside your vagina. (Clean yourselves off before having intercourse.)

Up the Ante

- Chew a few Altoids, or take a sip of schnapps, then explore your lover's backside and/or give him or her a rim job. If you want to intensify the sensation, introduce an ice cube for an unexpected combination of ice and spice.

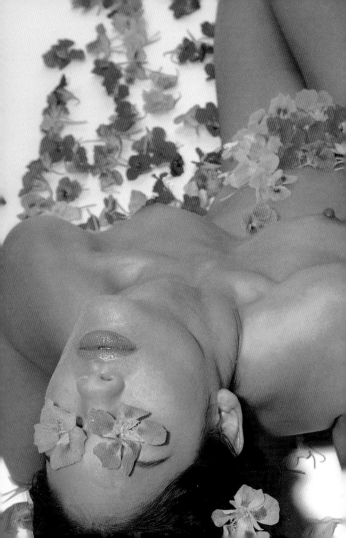

8

Bed of Flowers

Everyone loves getting flowers, but what about exploring your every fantasy in a bed of flowers? And did you know that certain flowers can be eaten right off your lover's body?

The Sexy Setup

Tell your lover you have a soft and sensuous game that's just right for a warm, sunny day in the garden.

Rules & Tools

If you can't find a bed of flowers for your game, you can make your own in a private spot outdoors. Simply purchase two dozen organically grown roses and take the flowers apart one by one to create a bed of petals. Other beautiful (and edible) flowers include organically grown violets and nasturtium (pictured). For the hot and spicy version of the game, be sure to bring along some honey.

Playing the Game

Sweet and safe: Disrobe your lover in a sensuous way, then have him or her lie down naked on the bed of flowers. Brush the blossoms or petals all over his or her body. Gently caress the base of the throat with the softest petals, then use the blossoms to trace a path from the throat to the nipples, belly, shoulders, buttocks, or thighs.

Hot and spicy: Create a ritual-like setting and adorn your lover's body with blossoms and petals, then add in swirls or dabs of honey. Tell her you're a bee looking for nectar and she must lie perfectly still while you eat, suck, or nibble the petals and honey away.

Up the Ante

- Hide the petals or blossoms in your crevices and ask your lover to eat his way out of the garden.

- Find a field of wildflowers and make love with full abandon. Only the birds will hear your cries of pleasure!

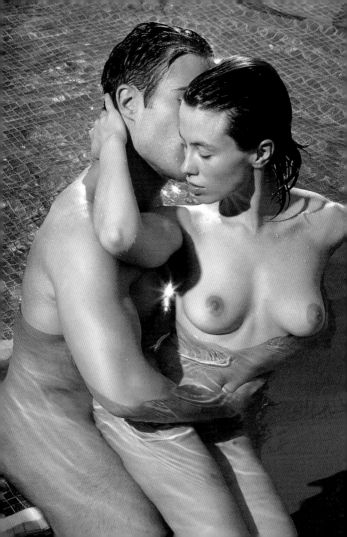

9

Poolside Pussy

Forget the images of screaming kids and lifeguards. These X-rated pool games are for adults only and best played under the stars.

The Sexy Setup

Tell your lover you have a nighttime poolside rendezvous planned, no bathing suit needed!

Rules & Tools

All you need is private and secluded access to a swimming pool and a clear, star-filled night for this naughty nighttime game.

Playing the Game

Sweet and safe: Try this erotic version of "Marco Polo" (bathing suit optional!). Hop into the pool and blindfold your lover. Tell him he must find you based on your moans of pleasure (loud for close, soft for far). Once he finds you, reward your lover with a wet and watery kiss, an underwater groping session, or a quick finger in the anus. Then switch roles!

Hot and spicy: Try some watery lovemaking positions using the pool to your advantage. Stay in the shallow end of the pool, and have your lover lean against the wall of the pool for added support. Wrap your legs around his waist and have him penetrate you. Hold on to the edge of the pool if needed. Alternatively, try the ladder: Face the ladder, holding the bars, and have your lover enter you from behind. Or try having him kneel on the step, and you straddle his lap.

Up the Ante

- Challenge your partner to fully remove his or her bathing suit in a public swimming pool and get it back on without anyone noticing.

- Sit naked at the very edge of the pool (or diving board, if he's really strong!) and have your lover pull himself up from underneath to lick and nuzzle your clitoris.

- Try making love on top of an inner tube, air mattress, or other floating pool toy!

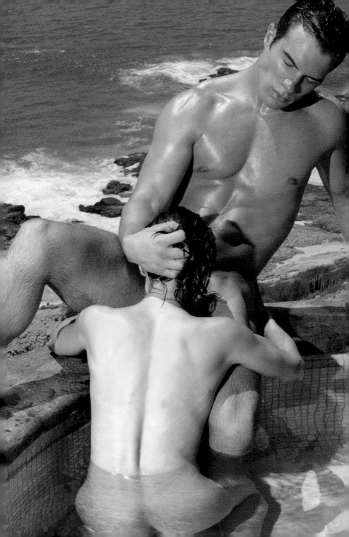

10

Hot Times in the Hot Tub

There's nothing like relaxing in a hot tub to soak away your worries, and everyone knows that a worry-free mind is open for naughty adventures.

The Sexy Setup

Tell your lover you have a nude party planned for the nearest hot tub, and there's one name on the invitation list: HIS!

Rules & Tools

Take care in the hot tub not to slip or submerge your head under water. Remember that water can dry out your genitals, so bring some lubricant along if needed.

Playing the Game

Sweet and safe: Ask your lover to sit on the bench, facing into the tub. Kneel on the bench, with your legs straddling him, before you lower yourself onto his penis. Hold on to the edge of the tub for better support as you raise and lower yourself.

Hot and spicy: Lower yourself onto your lover but face away from him, which will let him gently twist your nipples, stroke your clitoris, or massage your buttocks as you move up and down.

Up the Ante

- Kneel in front of a water jet so it stimulates your clitoris, then ask your lover to enter you from behind for double the fun!

- Have him sit or kneel in front of the water jet so it stimulates his anus. Kiss him passionately while you given him an underwater hand job.

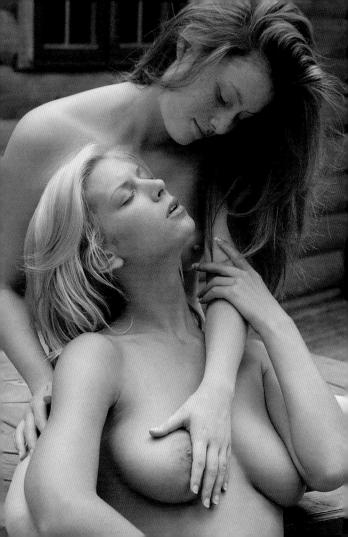

11

Playin' on the Playground

Think the playground is just for kids?
Think again! Swings, tunnels, and slides are the
perfect props for these adult-only games.

The Sexy Setup

Tell your lover to meet you at the playground after dark for some nighttime nooky.

Rules & Tools

Find a secluded and private playground. Bring flashlights, a bottle of wine, and blankets, if desired.

Playing the Game

Sweet and safe: Act like kids again, but this time do it in your birthday suits. Climb the ladder to the slide, pausing on the rung of your choice to give him a good look at your back side, then slide down the slide and have him kneel at the edge for some quick flicks of his tongue on your clitoris. Or, bring along a flashlight and play hide-and-seek in the dark (clothing optional!).

Hot and spicy: Have him sit on the swing, then you straddle him. Hold on tight! Alternatively, go through the tunnel slide together, side by side. When you get to the bottom, try making love inside the slide, or position yourself at the top of the tube and have him stand in front—your fully exposed genitals should be right at eye (and tongue!) level.

Up the Ante

- Have him tie you spread-eagle to the ladder rungs, then explore your every crevice with his hands and tongue. Alternatively, have him tie you backside facing out, then examine all your assets.

- Climb astride the overhead monkey bars with your legs over the bar and your genitals at face level. Ask him to explore your underside using his tongue, fingers, and hands!

- Sit in the swing and have him stimulate your clitoris with his tongue. Push away when the sensation is too strong, then swing back for more oral stimulation until you come!

- Try making love on a trampoline, in a tree house, or on the top bunk of a bunk bed! Remember, you *can* be a kid again when it comes to sexual adventure!

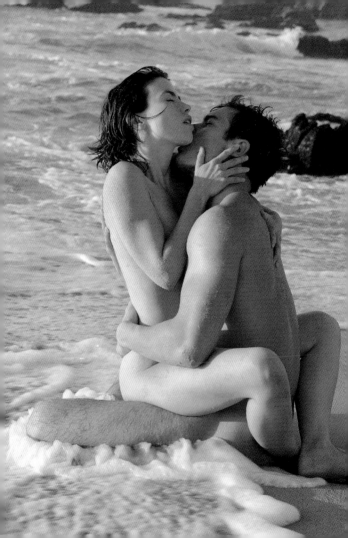

12

In the Lap of Luxury

This intimate and sexy position will surely bring you closer, both emotionally and sexually.

The Sexy Setup

Tell your lover you're in need of some full frontal nudity and contact, so be prepared for connecting your skin at every possible point. What's more, you'll do all the work while sitting on his lap.

Rules & Tools

All of these positions are done with both of you facing each other, so there's plenty of opportunity for making eye contact, licking his nipples, or having him fondle your breasts.

Playing the Game

Sweet and safe: Undress your lover in a slow and sensuous manner, then have him remove your clothing, all the while kissing your neck and breasts and rubbing his hands up and down your backside. Once you're both hot and wet, ask your lover to sit cross-legged. You should sit down on his lap, facing him, while inserting his penis into your vagina. Straddle his legs and wrap your legs around his back, then rub the front of your bodies together while you experience the sensations of shallow but tight penetration.

Hot and spicy: Lean back with one arm and hook one leg over his shoulder to change the angle of penetration, or slowly lean both arms backward, exposing your breasts for fondling or your clitoris for stimulation.

Up the Ante

- Ask your lover to stretch out his legs while you sit or lean back. To deepen the penetration, rest your legs on your partner's shoulders instead of wrapping them around his waist and lean back on your arms. For a sexy variation on this position that gives him full view of your naked torso, lie completely down on your back and lock your ankles behind his neck.

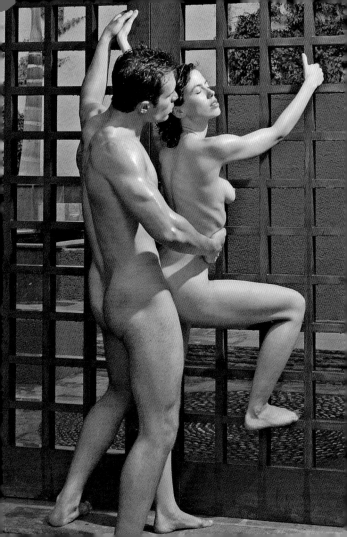

13

Prop Me Up
(and Drive It Home!)

This is the perfect sex game for locations where there's no room for lying down, such as a quickie in a restroom, a sexy encounter in the front hall, or a racy rendezvous in the closet while the kids watch a movie!

The Sexy Setup

Tell your lover you have a game that's sure to get a standing ovation. Mention that you've always wanted to enter her from behind, with her leg propped on a chair, or that you know a certain doorway that's perfect for face-to-face entry!

Rules & Tools

Bring along some lubrication, and perhaps a stool or chair for support.

Playing the Game

Sweet and safe: Undress each other slowly and sensuously, then find a place to prop your lover against the wall, facing away from you. Stroke her breasts and rub your hands down her belly, then slowly lift one of her legs up, prop it on a stool or small chair, and enter her from behind. The beauty of this position is that you can fondle her breasts, finger her clitoris, or gently bite the nape of her neck while you have intercourse!

Hot and spicy: Lean her against a wall or doorway, but have her face you so you can kiss her passionately, gently nip at her neck and shoulders, and run your hands down her backside. Lift one of her legs up, wrapping it around your waist or propping it on a small stool, then stoop slightly so you can enter her from below.

Up the Ante

- Brace yourself against a doorway with your hands on one side and your feet on the opposite side. Ask your lover to straddle you, with her feet on the same side of the doorway as you and her arms on the opposite side.

- Lean against the same doorpost, but invite your lover to climb aboard and hold on to your neck. Brace yourself with your legs while you thrust away!

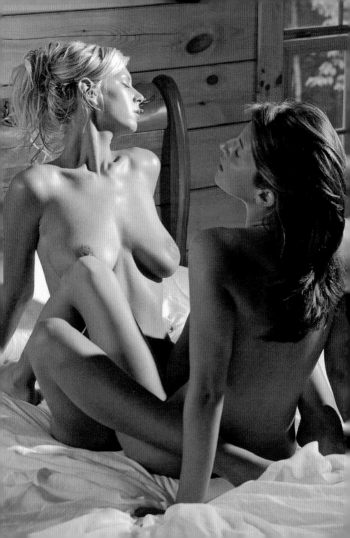

14

Scissors
of Love

This is a game designed for a pair of women,
but it can also be modified for you and
your male lover if it turns you on!

The Sexy Setup

Tell your female lover you're wondering what it will feel like to sit clit to clit, together! If your lover is male, tell him you have a jigsaw puzzle that needs assembling.

Rules & Tools

No real rules or tools here—just the desire to try a new and interesting position!

Playing the Game

Sweet and safe (for two women): Start things out slow, caressing each other, kissing, and gently removing each other's clothing. Once things are properly heated up (and you're both naked), move slowly into position: Scissor your legs, then scoot toward each other until your genitals touch. Gently bump and grind your genitals together for stimulation or orgasm; if you can't come without direct stimulation, unwind and take turns using your lips, tongue, or fingers to slowly caress and tease each other to orgasm.

Hot and spicy (for a man and a woman): Take your time with your foreplay, making sure your lover is rock hard before you move into position. Curl up on your side, exposing your genitals to your lover. He slides toward you, legs scissoring each other, in order to complete the jigsaw puzzle.

Up the Ante

- For two women: Try the male/female version of this position, but use a finger to stimulate your lover anally. Or, once she's in the curled position, take out your dildo and penetrate her while you rub together, clit to clit!

- While sitting in the sweet and safe position, insert a two-headed dildo into both of you and slide back and forth together.

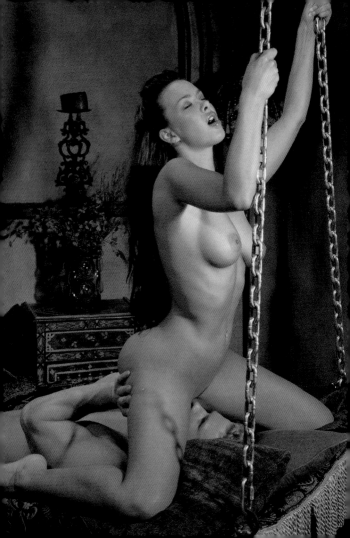

15

Sit on My Face

Come sit on my face—who hasn't heard that enticing line? Now you can turn it into a game that's sure to keep her coming back for more!

The Sexy Setup

Tell your lover you have a game where she gets to sit—right on the pleasure dome (your mouth)!

Rules & Tools

If you're not on a bed or other soft surface, put a blanket or pillow under her knees. Explain to her that she's in control—while you're there to pleasure her orally, she can control the intensity by moving up and down on your tongue. If she needs something to hold on to, position yourselves so she can lean her hands against the wall or hold on to the swing (as shown). For the hot and spicy version of the game, keep a butt plug or other anal device nearby.

Playing the Game

Sweet and safe: Have your lover kneel above your face, facing you, while you explore every inch of what's right in front of you. Start by kissing her inner thighs and taking in the smell and taste of her vulva. Give her genitals long, slow, and wet kisses, then introduce your tongue for exploring her labia, crevices, and clitoris. Find a rhythm she likes and bring her to a mind-blowing orgasm!

Hot and spicy: Have your lover kneel above your face, facing away from you, while you explore her genitals and backside. Use the same techniques as above, but don't restrict your kisses and tongue exploration to her labia and clitoris; run your tongue from her vagina to her anus and back again, all the while gently massing her buttocks. Put a finger or two inside her vagina and play with her G-spot, or introduce a butt plug or other anal device and insert that for triple stimulation!

Up the Ante

- Swap roles: Have her lie down, then kneel in front of her so your penis is right in front of her mouth (she may need a pillow or two to get the angle right). Have her hold your penis with one hand and explore your backside with the other; she might fondle your testicles, insert a finger into your anus, or just lightly trace her fingertips along your perineum.

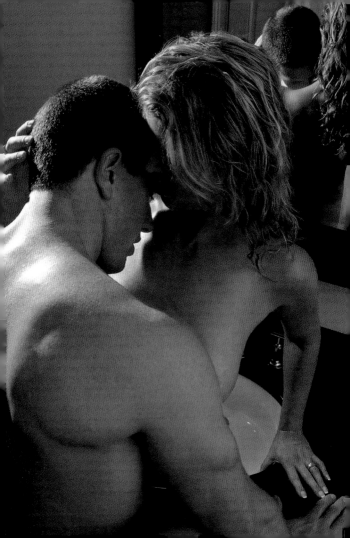

16

Restroom Rendezvous

Off to the museum, watching a ball game, or stuck at a conference all day? What better place for some quick and excitlng sex than the local restroom?

The Sexy Setup

If you and your lover are attending a conference, but
listening to different sessions, send him a text message
telling him you have something burning hot to talk to him
about. Wandering through the museum together? Lean
into him suggestively, letting your breast rub against his
upper arm, and tell him to meet you in the last stall of the
women's room at a certain time.

Rules & Tools

Time is of the essence with this game, so get yourself
stimulated before your lover appears. Remember, if anyone
looks under the door to see whether the stall is occupied,
only one pair of shoes can show—preferably those of the
appropriate sex!

Playing the Game

Sweet and safe: In the women's room: Have your lover stand on the toilet seat and let his pants slide off, presenting his penis right at your mouth level. Run your tongue up his thighs, fondle his buttocks, and cup his testicles in your hands. Once he's rock hard, give him a blow job or bring him to orgasm by hand, but be sure to catch his come in your mouth or a handful of tissue paper before you flush.

Hot and spicy: In the men's room: Remove your underclothes, then stand on the toilet seat, but raise one foot up onto the toilet paper holder to give him full access to your genitals. Hold the top of the stall or put your hands on the ceiling for extra support. Have your lover explore your thighs, labia, and clitoris with his tongue or insert a few fingers into your vagina or anus. Remember to keep your moans to a minimum if he brings you to orgasm.

Up the Ante

- Try having sex in a porta potty or in the restroom at a bar, a club, a restaurant, or an airport.

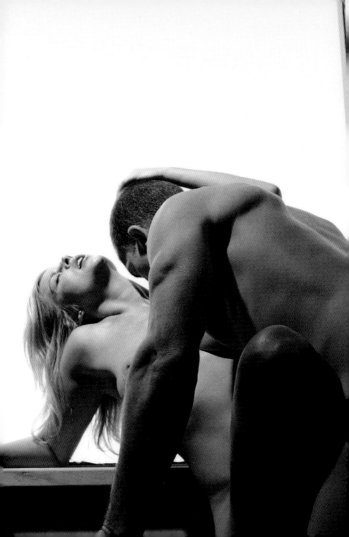

17

Mile High Club

Who hasn't heard of the Mile High Club, or the "secret" society of couples who've had sex on an airplane? Now it's your turn to join this sexy sect!

The Sexy Setup

This is a good game for surprising your lover, but if she doesn't like surprises you can start this game right in your seat, either by whispering suggestive ideas into her ear or fondling her thighs under the blanket.

Rules & Tools

You can try this game on just about any flight, but a red-eye flight (where the plane is flying overnight) is often the best choice, because most of the other passengers will be sleeping. If you get caught in the restroom, tell the other passengers or the flight attendant that your partner got sick and you were helping her out.

Playing the Game

Sweet and safe: Use this game as foreplay for meeting in the restroom, or bring each other to orgasm without leaving your seats. You'll need a blanket for covering your genitals. Start by kissing your lover's neck, then fondle her breasts. Ask her to slip off her panties and spread her legs so you can finger her to orgasm. To reciprocate, ask her to go down on you with the blanket over her head.

Hot and spicy: Head to the restroom separately. Work out a special knock so you can let her in once she arrives. There are plenty of different positions to try out, so this is a game that you can play over and over. Have your lover lean against the sink so you can enter her doggie style, sit on the sink and wrap her legs around your waist, or put one foot up on the toilet and enter her from behind. Prefer a seated position? Put the toilet seat down and sit on the seat, then have her climb on top facing the door. Fondle her breasts and hold on tight in case of unexpected turbulence!

Up the Ante

- Once you get home, play the "Flirty Flight Attendant" role-play game, #20.

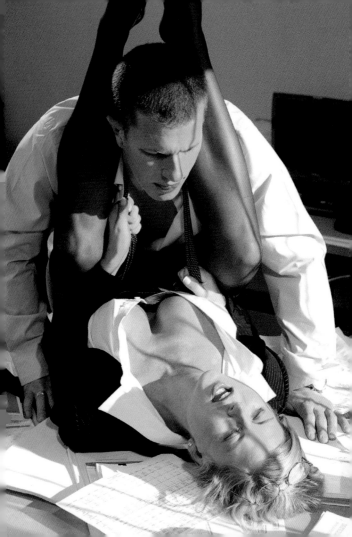

18

Hold My Calls
(and My Balls!)

Sometimes a man just can't wait till he gets
home for a taste of his lover. There's no need to
wait all day with this naughty office game!

The Sexy Setup

Call your lover and ask her if she's got a few minutes for a quick lunch or if you can meet her at her office after hours. Set a time you're going to meet, and mention that you're bringing a friend (use your favorite pet name for your penis).

Rules & Tools

If this is a daytime encounter, make sure you've scoped out her office ahead of time for empty closets, dead-end stairwells, offices that lock, or unused conference rooms. Bring along lubrication and plan a time when most people are out of the office, such as lunchtime or during a special meeting.

Playing the Game

Sweet and safe: Greet your lover with a passionate kiss, then lead her to the dead-end stairwell. Open her blouse and kiss, fondle, and tease her breasts, neck, and shoulders until she's wet, then lean her against the wall and enter her from behind or prop her on the stair railing and have her wrap her legs around your waist.

Hot and spicy: Tell her you'd really like to see her office. Once you're in, quickly close the door and lock it. Kiss her passionately while reaching under her skirt and pulling her panties down. Back her slowly up to her desk, clear off any critical papers, and lift her up onto the desk. Spread her legs and enter her standing up, with her vagina right at the edge of the desk, or lay her down and squeeze her nipples while you thrust away.

Up the Ante

- To up the thrill factor, seek out semiprivate areas for hot and steamy sex: a darkened corner of the corporate library, under the conference room table, or in the utility or coat closet. You can even lift her onto a copy machine, lay her on a lunchroom table, or do her on the waiting room couch!

- To heighten the excitement, add in a boss/secretary role-playing game.

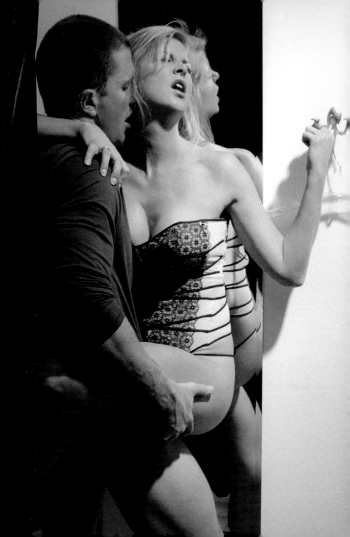

19

The Un-Dressing Room

This is a game that's fun for both parties—
you get some new clothes and some
sexual satisfaction in the same day!

The Sexy Setup

Tell your lover you'd like to go shopping, but you need him to rate your outfits. Mention that you're planning to model a number of different ensembles, from full-length gowns to lingerie and bathing suits.

Rules & Tools

Scout out the stores ahead of time to locate the least-visited or most private dressing rooms. Plan to visit the store when it's not too busy, such as in the evening, an hour before closing, or other off hours. (Of course, if you're feeling really daring you can try this game on a weekend afternoon, a national day off from work, or right around the holidays when the stores tend to be busiest!)

Playing the Game

Sweet and safe: Stroll around the store together, arm in arm, looking at clothing, lingerie, dresses, and even shoes and hats. Ask him what colors and fabrics he likes, or what style of things he'd like to see you model. If possible, really reach outside your comfort zone and pick out some sexy, suggestive, or even slutty clothing. The hotter the better!

Take the clothing back to the dressing room, and find him a seat just outside the dressing room. One by one, model the outfits, taking your time to turn slowly, flash him some leg or breast, or just come close to him. Make sure you ask him which outfit he likes the best, and buy that one for additional fun later on!

Hot and spicy: If your sweet and safe game is really turning him on, invite him into the dressing room. Ask him to help you put on his favorite outfit by zipping you in or fastening your buttons. As his fingers do the work, ask him to stop at certain places and explore. Give him a couple of hot, passionate kisses and some gentle groping to get him hard, then slip off the garments and have sex against the wall, on the dressing room floor, or even on the little seat. Use the mirror for added stimulation!

Up the Ante

- Wear your sexy outfit over to the men's dressing rooms. Make sure you flash a few of the other men or flirt with your eyes; your lover will enjoy knowing he's got you all to himself while surrounded by other men.

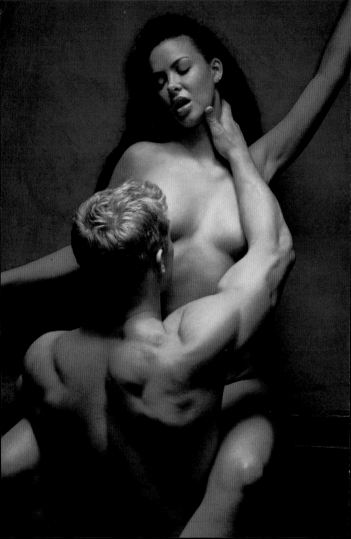

20

Flirty Flight Attendant

This is a good game for women who like to be dominant and men who like taking orders from a woman in charge!

The Sexy Setup

Tell your lover you have a naughty game where he's the passenger and you're the flirty flight attendant who's going to teach him a lesson about proper in-flight conduct.

Rules & Tools

Set up the scene beforehand. Dress in your sexiest flight attendant outfit, complete with stockings, heels, and lingerie. Have some props on hand, such as a drink tray, cups, peanuts, and napkins, as well as a small pillow, a blanket, an eye cover (the kind they give out on overnight flights), and a pair of handcuffs. Next, find a chair in your house that resembles an airline seat and prepare for take-off!

Playing the Game

Sweet and safe: Have your lover play airplane traveler by asking for food or drinks, but then do things by "accident" to upset you. He can spill his drink, ask for multiple pillows, etc. When you get annoyed, have him try to kiss you or touch you inappropriately (and keep trying). Once you're completely fed up, tell him you're going to restrain him—then pull out a pair of cuffs and fasten his hands behind him.

Now it's your turn to take the game wherever you want by teasing him with a flash of your breasts, man-handling him until he's hard, or demanding he follow your every command and satisfy you *now*!

Hot and spicy: Follow the same game as above, but step it up a notch on the bossy (or bitchy) scale. When he spills his drink, lean across him in a bossy manner and accidentally bump your breasts into his face; if he tries to kiss you, push him around or slap him gently. When he asks for more drinks or pillows, alternate between acting put out and being ready to put out. Remove your stockings in a teasing manner, making sure he gets a good view of your thighs and genitals, and then use the stockings to tie him to the chair. Begin your punishment by undressing him from the waist down, then teasing him using your hands, mouth, and lips. Each time he seems ready to orgasm, pull away. Once you're hot and wet, climb on him and take him to new heights of passion!

Up the Ante

- Before you restrain him, get into a gentle struggle (but let him win). Have him tie you to the chair, then either tease you into submission or take you forcibly while you fight back.

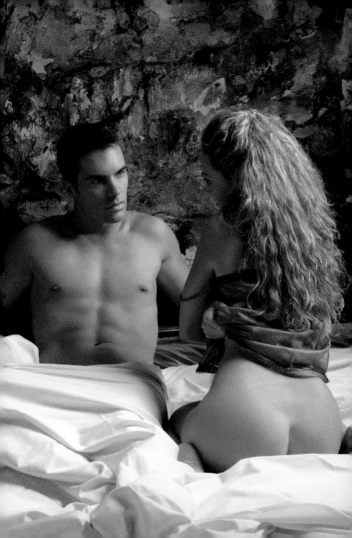

21

Horny Housemaid

Here's a great game for the man who likes to be serviced—and a woman who likes to take care of her man.

The Sexy Setup

Ask your lover to come home, put his feet up, and relax.
Make him a drink or serve him some appetizers, then tell
him you have a little game in mind that's sure to perk
him up!

Rules & Tools

For the sweet and safe game, pull your hair back in a slop-
py bun and dress in a dowdy housedress (but wear sizzling
hot lingerie underneath and be prepared to shake out your
hair). For the hot and spicy game, buy a true French maid
uniform complete with white cap and gloves, tiny apron,
short skirt, and feather duster (undergarments optional!).

Playing the Game

Sweet and safe: Come into the room in a shy and
reserved way and start tidying up, but glance his way to
see if he's watching you. There are two options: Really
draw out the submissive act, moving suggestively around
the room, then suddenly strip off the housedress, shake out
your hair, and pounce on him. Or remove the outfit piece
by piece in a seductive striptease, emerging at the end as a
tempting temptress ready to clean his house!

Hot and spicy: Pretend he's the overworked, lonesome bachelor who's relaxing with his favorite drink—and getting ready to watch an adult film. Knock on the door and call out, "Maid service, may I come in?" Start tidying up the room, making sure you lean over suggestively, flashing him a peak under your skirt. Sit next to him and ask if there's anything that needs special attention—after all, you're at his service and you aim to please. Perhaps he needs help undressing so you can do the laundry, or would he like you to turn on the movie for him? Take off his clothes and leave the room, then come back suddenly (and catch him masturbating). Tell him that's your job, and take over with your hands, mouth, and lips. Make sure you clean up any extra mess you make!

Up the Ante

- Play a game of "Masturbating Maid." Tie him up with your apron and tease or tickle him with your feather duster. Once he's tied up, slowly undress yourself, stroking your nipples, caressing your breasts, and fingering your clitoris. Bring yourself to climax while he's tied down and forced to watch, then ask him how you can be of *service*!

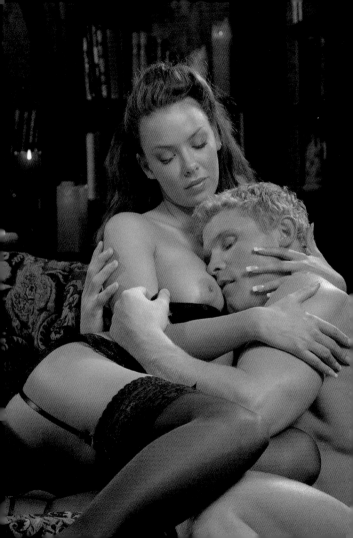

22

Pirate and Captive Maiden

You can play your own version of Captain
Jack Sparrow with this role-playing game—
just get ready to capture the bootie!

The Sexy Setup

Tell your lover you have a swashbuckling game in mind: You're going to be the pirate and she gets to play the captive maiden. If she's willing, ask her to dress in a maiden's outfit, like a dress with a low-cut top, plenty of jewelry, and a full skirt (with no undergarments!).

Rules & Tools

You need to dress like a pirate for this game, whether that means buying a costume or making your own. Take your inspiration from books and movies: Wrap your head in a bandanna, darken your eyes, put on a big white shirt unbuttoned to your waist, slip into your tightest pants, and put on your seafaring boots. Collect your props, such as an eye patch, a hook for a hand, or a toy parrot on your shoulder.

Playing the Game

Sweet and safe: Open the game with this line: "Ahoy, mates! Keep your hands off the Captain's maiden!" Then pretend you're protecting her from a room full of leering faces and dozens of hands by pulling her onto your lap, stroking her hair, and kissing her bosom.

Reach under her skirt and secretly pleasure her while the other pirates continue drinking, eating, and making noise. She's your captive, but you're her protector!

Hot and spicy: This time she's your captive, but you're the horny pirate who's been at sea far too long. It's been months since you've seen a woman, let alone touched one, and she's beautiful to boot. Tie her hands behind her back and manhandle her breasts, or rip off her dress and tie her naked to a chair for your viewing pleasure. Tease her breasts and nipples with your lips and mouth until she's wet, then pull her hair and kiss her roughly. Take her any way you want—you're the captain of this boat!

Up the Ante

- If your lover is willing, make her your sex slave. Rip her clothes off, then make her perform all the duties of a captive maiden completely naked. That might include hoisting the sails (removing your clothing), walking the plank (sucking you off), and swabbing the deck (cleaning up the mess!).

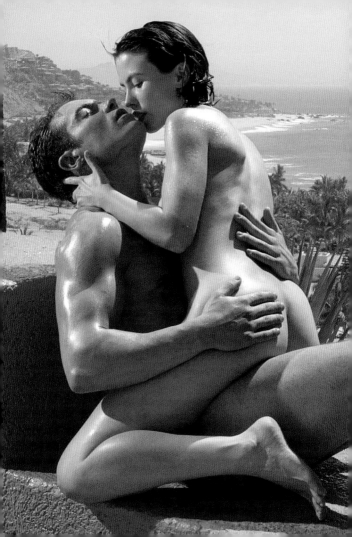

23

Mistress (or Master) and Sex Slave

Do you love the idea of having your own personal sex slave? Do you tingle at the thought of ordering your lover to pleasure you whenever you want? Then this is the game for you.

The Sexy Setup

Tell your lover that you have a game he's sure to love (especially if he likes being dominated). Tell him you're the beautiful princess, and he's the handsome sex slave who must do (or wear) whatever his mistress desires.

Rules & Tools

Dress in your favorite princess outfit: Put on your sexiest bikini-style top, bikini bottoms (preferably with an attached loincloth), and decorative belt, choker, and armbands. Dress your lover in a loincloth or nothing at all. Assemble a pair of handcuffs, choker, or other props as desired.

Playing the Game

Sweet and safe: Order your lover to give you pleasure, whether that means feeding you by hand, massaging your feet, or brushing your hair. If you want him to caress your breasts, suck your nipples, or squeeze your butt, order him to do so until you want him to stop. Direct him to all your favorite spots, and order him to do whatever feels good for you. Remember, this is all about your pleasure—and as slave, he must do whatever his mistress wants.

Hot and spicy: Swap roles, and ask him to handcuff your hands together. Now you're his sex slave, and he's the master. He can order you to lick his entire body, let him penetrate you anally, or he can expose parts of you for his own pleasure—he's in control.

Up the Ante

- Buy your lover a choker and leash and lead him from room to room like a dog. When you want pleasure, tell him to do it (or face punishment). Keep a paddle or crop on hand for punishing his failure to pleasure you completely or showing any sign of disrespect.

- Take it outside: Make your lover go places in public without undergarments or masturbate in a public place (while you watch). Remember, you're in charge!

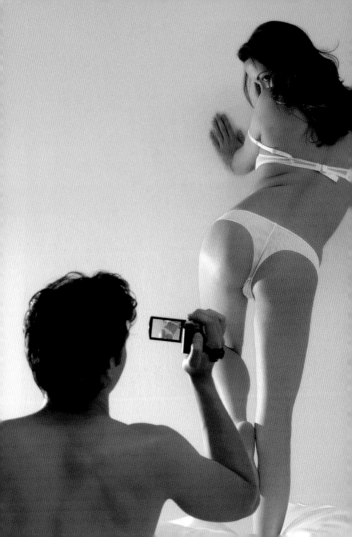

24

Porn Star and Director

This is a fun game for either partner—
one gets to be the budding porn star
(or centerfold model) while the other
person plays director. Roll the cameras!

The Sexy Setup

Tell your lover you want her to play the budding center-fold and/or porn star, and you're the director of the photo shoot. As a virgin to the industry, she must follow your every command.

Rules & Tools

Set up a sexy area for her photo shoot, such as a fur-covered couch, a bed with silk sheets, or a bearskin rug in front of the fire. Keep different props and sex toys nearby (hot and spicy). Ask her to dress in her sexiest lingerie or bikini, but to wear a short robe over her outfit.

Load your camera with film (or charge your digital camera) and/or set up your camcorder or handheld video camera. Dress like this is all business. If you really want your photos to look authentic, buy a few porn magazines ahead of time and study the photos.

Playing the Game

Sweet and safe: Have your lover pose for her centerfold shots, but tell her it's all about looking sensuous and sexy. You can direct her to remove her clothing, fondle herself, lean over suggestively, lie on her stomach and expose her buttocks, or pull her lingerie aside to expose her genitals. Take photos of each pose, then organize them into a slide-show and watch it together.

Hot and spicy: Tell your lover this photo shoot is for a true porn magazine, and she has to do whatever turns you on (even if she objects)—pinch her own nipples, finger herself, or wear handcuffs so you can insert a butt plug or dildo (and then take pictures). Now's the time to pose her in the way you've always imagined her, or to ask her to act out *your* favorite fantasies!

Up the Ante

- Get out the camcorder or video camera and shoot a movie, such as *Naughty Nympho* or *I Can't Stop Masturbating*. Give your lover her lines, direct her moves, and film away!

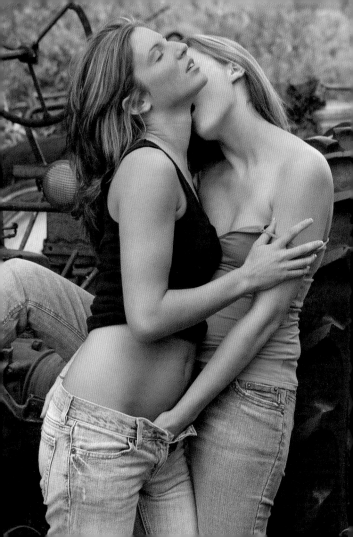

25

Farm Girl in the Hay

Every man fantasizes about a romp in the clover with the lonely farm girl or a quickie in the hay with the milkmaid. Here's your chance to act out that fantasy in the privacy of your own home.

The Sexy Setup

Tell your lover you have a game to play, then describe one of the roles for you (and one for him) as detailed below.

Rules & Tools

Pick a role: the innocent virgin farm girl who needs sex instruction, the naughty milkmaid who likes nooky in the hay, or the quiet, shy girl next door who's really a vixen at heart. Arrange a date and time for him to come visit you, and give him a role to play: the experienced farmhand, the farmer's shy and timid son, or the horny teenager next door who masturbates every night.

Playing the Game

Sweet and safe: If you're the innocent virgin farm girl, dress in overalls, with a tiny top underneath. Put your hair in pigtails and tie a bandanna around your neck (this might come in handy later for light bondage). Then tell your lover (the experienced farmhand) to pretend he's teaching you the ins and outs of sex: where he likes to be touched or kissed, where he wants to kiss or touch you, and so on. Let him lead the way, and really try to pretend like you've never done this before.

Hot and spicy: This time, you play the naughty milk-maid, and he plays the farmer's shy and timid son. Dress the part of a milkmaid (think flowered dress and no undergarments) or the farm girl (overalls with nothing underneath). You lead him by the hand and show him all the details of the birds and the bees.

Up the Ante

- You play the role of the shy girl next door, and he plays the part of the horny teenager. Pretend you're shy and timid while he tries hard to seduce you. At some point in the game, drop the shy role and turn on your inner vixen!

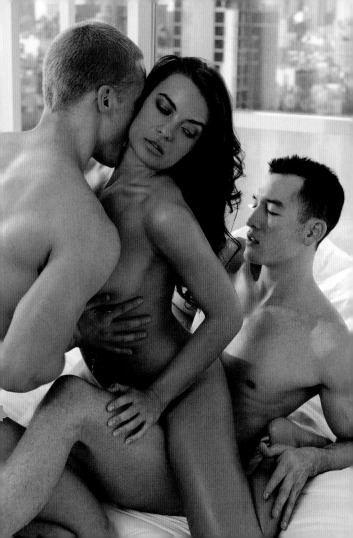

26

Oreo Cookie
(and You're the Filling!)

This game is designed for two men and one
woman. The idea: sandwich her from either side
like an Oreo cookie, and she's the yummy filling!

The Sexy Setup

Tell your lover that you want to maximize her pleasure—
you and another male friend are going to worship her body
and give her all the pleasure she can take.

Rules & Tools

This is a game designed for pleasuring the female; it's perfect for women who aren't that comfortable with sexual
contact between two men. Decide which of you wants to
"service" her front side, and which of you wants to play
"backdoor man."

Playing the Game

Sweet and safe: This is a simple game of two on one.
She sits back and does nothing but orgasm, while you two
sandwich her from either side. Start by undressing her
with one of you facing her front (and kissing her passionately), while the other works from the rear. As you undress
her, focus on her front side—touch her breasts, nuzzle her
neck, and kiss her belly. Your backside partner should do
the same: Kiss the small of her back, fondle her backside,
and caress her thighs.

Ultimately, the front side lover should manually or orally stimulate her clitoris in order to bring her to orgasm while the backside partner spoons her from behind, fondles her from behind, and squeezes her nipples. Having two sets of hands all over her body is sure to drive her crazy!

Hot and spicy: Turn up the action. While you kiss and fondle her from the front side, have your backside partner enter her from behind. Once he's thrusting in and out, move down and stimulate her clitoris orally. She won't know whether she's coming or going!

Up the Ante

- Stimulate her orally, but have your backside partner stimulate her anus with a set of anal beads.

- For the ultimate four-prong orgasm, kiss her deeply while stimulating her clitoris manually. Have your backside partner enter her from behind and insert a finger into her anus. Every orifice accounted for!

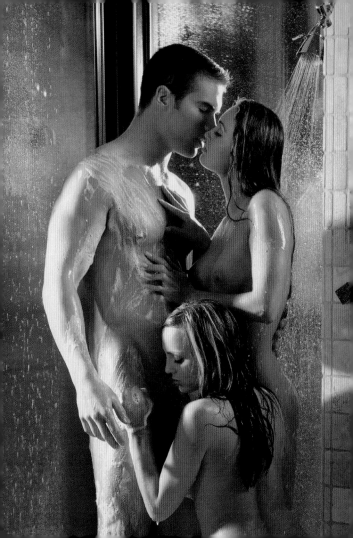

27

Merry Go Round

Here's a game where everybody's giving—
and receiving—pleasure. It works best
for two women and a male lover, but you can
switch to two men and a woman
if everyone's comfortable.

The Sexy Setup

Tell your female lover you want to hook up with her and one of her sexiest friends (she can pick who she wants to join you). Then ask if she prefers to be a giver or a taker—either role is fine with you.

Rule & Tools

There are two roles in this game: the lover who gives pleasure, and the lover who receives it. The goal is to have everyone playing both roles at once.

Playing the Game

Sweet and safe: Take turns kissing, touching, and undressing among the three of you until everyone is naked. Then suggest you all take a shower together, where the steam and heat can help everyone relax. Stand up, kiss your female lover, and finger her clitoris while her girlfriend sucks on you and masturbates at the same time. Alternatively, have your lover stand up while you kiss her genitals and clitoris; she can kiss and finger her girlfriend while you masturbate.

Hot and spicy: Move to the bed for this action. Lie down, and ask your female lover to sit on your face, facing your feet. Have her girlfriend climb on you cowgirl style. You stimulate your lover orally while the two girls kiss and fondle each other's breasts. The second woman rides you to orgasm!

Up the Ante

- Have one of the two female lovers lie down. Kneel over her in a classic 69 so she can suck you off. You stimulate the second woman orally while she fingers her girlfriend's clitoris!

- Let everyone find a penis or clitoris to touch, suck, lick, and stimulate—then try to orgasm simultaneously!

The Publisher maintains the records relating to images in
this book required by 18 USC 2257. Records are located at
Quarto Publishing Group USA Inc., 100 Cummings Center,
Suite 406-L, Beverly, MA 01915-6101.

19 18 17 16 15   4 5

ISBN: 978-1-59233-668-5

Cover design by traffic
Photography by Allan Penn Photography

Printed and bound in Hong Kong